Other books by Susan Hawthorne

Fiction
The Falling Woman (1992)

Poetry
"The Language in My Tongue", in *Four New Poets* (1993)

Non-fiction
The Spinifex Quiz Book (1993)

Anthologies (poetry, fiction, drama)
Difference (1985)
Moments of Desire (with Jenny Pausacker, 1989)
The Exploding Frangipani (with Cathie Dunsford, 1990)
Angels of Power (with Renate Klein, 1991)
Car Maintenance, Explosives and Love (with Cathie Dunsford and
    Susan Sayer, 1997)

Anthologies (non-fiction)
Australia for Women (with Renate Klein, 1994)
CyberFeminism (with Renate Klein, 1999)

SUSAN HAWTHORNE

Bird

AND OTHER WRITINGS ON EPILEPSY

SPINIFEX

Spinifex Press Pty Ltd
504 Queensbury Street
North Melbourne, Vic. 3051
Australia
women@spinifexpress.com.au
http://www.spinifexpress.com.au/~women

First edition published by Spinifex Press, 1999.

Typeset in Garamond 10.5pt on 13 by Sandra Goldbloom Zurbo
Cover design by Deb Snibson, Modern Art Productions
Made and printed in Australia by Australian Print Group

National Library of Australia
Cataloguing-in-Publication data:

Hawthorne, Susan, 1951-
   Bird and other writings on epilepsy

   ISBN 1 875559 88 4
   1. Epilepsy - Poetry. I. Title.

A821.3

For the friends who've sat with me.

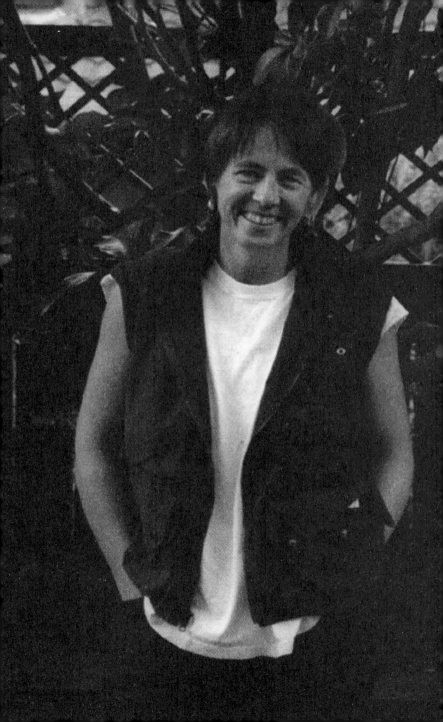

Contents

BIRD

i

I want to be a bird. I know that sounds silly,
but it's a metaphor. When I say I want to be
a bird, what I mean is that I want to be
a trapeze artist. Fly through the air, spin and twirl
and catch on to the bar again.

I know I could do it. I can swing from my legs,
I can hang upside down for hours—well almost.
I can stand on my hands and my head
I'm learning how to do somersaults in the air.
My teacher told me that back somersaults are easier
because you can see where you're going.
I believe her.
I can do it in my head. And Ms Quick is always
right about these things.
She was right about putting your hands in
a triangle for a headstand.

I can do a back dive into the pool. Straight over.
I can't do a back walkover yet, but some day I'll get it.
Amy's the only one who can do them, but
she started gymnastics when she was seven.
She's neater, but I can do a handspring with more oomph.

At dinner tonight I was talking and Mum
said I shouldn't get too serious. I looked at
her and couldn't figure out why she said that.

I was doing my homework when she came in. She said

I shouldn't get too serious about gymnastics and aerials,
it could be dangerous.

Mum,
I said,
just because I'm a girl it doesn't mean
I can't do these things.

It's not that. Girls can do anything.
It's the fits.

The fits again, oh jesus.
The little turns,
she used to call them,
now it's the fits.

If you have one when you're high up
you could injure yourself seriously.
You might not be able to walk again.

Mum,
I just want to learn the trapeze.
I don't want to go sky diving.
One day you might.

Sure, but that's not now.
Look Mum, I'll be careful.
Truly.
I wouldn't do it if I felt funny.
You promise?
Yeah, I promise.
It took the wind out of me a bit.

ii

I forgot to tell you my name.
It's Avis.
I used to feel strange having the same
name as hire cars, but it's a real word.
Latin for bird.
Isn't that great?

iii

I stood and waited at the bus stop
for a long time today. It just didn't come.
So I was late for school.
When I said the bus was late, some smart alec
yelled out that the bus driver tooted at me
and when I didn't move he drove off.
I can't figure it out. I know the bus didn't come.

iv

My best friend's name is Gabriella. We talk a lot.
I said I didn't believe what Jenny said
about my late excuse. The bus just didn't come.
She believes me.

v

I had a funny dream last night. I was at this really old place,
a building with turrets. I was standing on the turrets
and someone asked me to jump. I wasn't scared at all and
when I jumped, I flew. Someone was holding on to my feet
and we were flying ten metres above the ground.
I can still feel it, the air supporting me.
It's much easier to fly than I thought.

vi

I told Gabriella about my dream
she just raised her eyebrows and said, Sure,
it's easy in dreams. Then she said,
But if you tried it in real life you'd break your neck.
She knows how I feel about learning the trapeze,
but she's not interested at all.
She'd rather read maths text books.
Weird. But we're best friends all the same.

vii

After sports class we had to "play with the computers".
Gabriella shows me cool tricks now and then. Her Dad's
a computer salesman so she knows all these things.
Today, when no one was watching, while we were "playing",
she showed me how we could look up our marks and
files on the school computer. I stood guard
while she hacked her way in.

We were browsing the files for our names—and there they were.
Our last names are next to one another on the roll—
that's how we got to be friends—and then she said
Look you've got a thick one there. And before I knew it
we were looking at my medical history. It said in great big letters,
EPILEPSY.
Grand mal and petit mal, it said.

Gabriella looked at me like a fish.
I didn't know what to say. So I didn't say anything.
She had a good long read. I was trying to skim ahead

to see if it said something awful that I didn't want her to read.
But there wasn't much there really
a couple of instances of staring
and the pills I take.
So what, I thought.

viii
How come you didn't tell me? she said that afternoon.
I didn't think it was too important.
Yes you do. I saw your face.
It is important and you didn't trust me enough to tell me.
It's not true. It's nice not to have to think about it.
At home, it's in the air in everything I do.
I catch Mum watching me secretly. She thinks I don't notice.
And she's always saying, Have you had your pills? or,
Don't stare, or . . . well, just something that makes me know
she's thinking about the fits again.
It's not that I didn't . . . don't trust you.
I just wanted time away from it. You know?
Yeah, okay.

ix
Things changed a little after that.
It wasn't all that noticeable, but I noticed it.
I'd catch Gabriella at Mum's trick:
watching. Still, we stayed best friends.

x
The trapeze Ms Quick's been talking about went up today.
I was so excited I said, Oh, Ms Quick, you're really. . .

you're the best teacher in the school.
Gabriella was sitting next to me, cringing.
But I didn't care.

xi

Mum didn't seem to understand why I was so happy.
I even got into bed before she told me to tonight.
I'm so happy. I just want to go to sleep
so I can wake up and get to our class tomorrow.

xii

I'm on stage. It's a huge auditorium.
Bigger than the school hall. And old.
It has decorative things on the walls and
lamps and a beautiful red velvet curtain
across the stage. There are boxes for
the special people to sit in. But tonight
they're empty because that's where my
trapeze goes. I am swinging wildly
across the stage. I have to be able to let go
and fly from one box to the other and land
perched on the edge like a bird.
I'm swinging my last time and I let go.
I'm flying across the stage. Up higher.
I can hear the people holding their breath
below me. And then it happens.
I begin to fall. I scream and scream . . .
and Mum's there asking what the matter is. I
don't want to tell her but I'm too scared not to.

xiii

Mum didn't say anything to me this morning.
Just looked. Looked like she was walking
around in my skull with a torch.

xiv

I changed as quick as I could and
was down in the gym waiting.
Gabriella yelled, Wait for me.
But I couldn't.
I'll wait for you down there.
And I ran off.

There it was, swinging just slightly.
Maybe someone came in and pushed it.
My fingers can just touch the bar.
The others came in and stood looking at it
like it was some kind of torture machine.
Then Ms Quick came in.

We had to warm up first. I just wanted
to run over and swing on it. But I controlled myself
and laughed as I watched Gabriella cheat her way
through the warm ups.

Who would like to have a go at the trapeze today?
My hand shot up. A couple of other hands crawled
in the air and Amy's too. We had to wait while
she got the others going on something that
didn't need her watching. And then she came back.
There were just five of us.

First thing, she said, is to make sure you never
go on this alone. Make sure there are always two catchers
with you. I wasn't sure I wanted to be friends with this lot,
but I guessed I'd have to.

She leapt up and grabbed the bar.
Her body was so straight.
Without swinging she lifted her body towards the bar.
She did this three times, then swung her legs up,
tucked her toes in and hung upside down.
She was so relaxed. Then she swung her legs
straight back over her head in a jack-knife,
held it for a moment and then her feet were
between her arms and on the ground.

Avis? she said, with hardly a questioning tone.
I leapt for the bar and grabbed it.
I was halfway into getting up so I could
hang by my legs when she said, Not so fast.
She had me doing chin-ups. They were hard.
She had to help me.
It looked so easy when she did it.
Now, she said, can you hang from your knees?
I got my legs up, then I let go
and felt my body swing down, arms wide open,
just like a bird.

Amy had a go next. She was so neat.
But she's shorter than me and had to be helped
to reach the bar. We watched as she moved

around the bar like a monkey. I didn't know
you could do half those things. But she's good.
I'll have to practise. Then the others had a go.
Luisa's taller than me and just held on to the bar.
She hooked her toes in and got her legs through.
She hung like a sloth, four limbs curled around
the branch. She wouldn't let go her hands.
Ms Quick cajoled her and held on, but she didn't look right.
All crooked. Then it was Sharon's turn.
She just hung by her hands and squirmed as
Ms Quick lifted her, heaved her into pull-ups.
Mandy just shook her head when it came to her turn.
Nah, she said. It doesn't look safe to me, and turned away.

xv

Every Wednesday after school, Ms Quick stays back
and we have trapeze classes. Four of us turn up
most weeks. I can do a whole lot more things now:
bird's nests and even hanging by an arm and a leg.
What I like best is falling from a bluebird -
that's when you balance on the bar across your tummy
and stay there, arms wide. When you fall
you pull your legs wider so they catch hold
of the ropes and you just hang there, comfortable.
It's the falling that feels so good.

xvi

Gabriella stayed behind this afternoon to watch.
When we got on the bus she said, You've gotten really good.
How do you do it? Aren't you scared?

Nup, I said. It makes me fearless.
I feel like that's what I'm meant to do.
You know how when you're sitting at a computer
and you just know what to do next, because it's in
your blood or something, it's the same.
I just know what to do. And if it doesn't work,
I have another go. I know I'm not as good as Amy,
but it doesn't excite her as much. It's just one more thing
she's good at. For me, it's like food.
She nodded and looked out the window for a while.

What about . . . ? You know, your epilepsy?
Doesn't that make it dangerous for you?
I could feel my hair climbing up my neck.
Why would it? I don't have fits much and anyway,
if I do it's always in the morning or during the night.
It's not a problem. Okay?
All right. I was just worried, that's all.
Her stop was next.
I sat there staring out the window, watching
the birds fly between electric wires, landing
on roof tops and perching on poles.
Why don't they just leave me alone?

xvii
The worst thing ever happened today.
I was in the gym and one of the girls hurt herself,
sprained her ankle, so they called Mrs Miller down.
She does all the first aid stuff. There I was
hanging beautifully from the trapeze,
getting more and more agile and skilful.

She looked at me with horror in her eyes
as she struggled out with the limping girl.
When I got back to the classroom there was a message:
I should go to the staffroom to see her.

I knocked and she came out.
Avis, she said, I'm going to have to stop you
from doing tricks on the trapeze.
You know, it could be very dangerous
for someone like you.

I screamed.
Screamed in my heart and
squeezed my lips tight so
nothing would come out.

I said with all the control I could muster,
No you won't,
and spun round and walked away.
War.
It was war between me and Mrs Miller.

xviii
Ms Quick looked strangely at me next time.
I knew Mrs Miller had been in her ear.
She beckoned me over to her.
Avis, is it true . . . that you have epilepsy?
I nodded, although I meant to shake my head
and say no.
This makes it very hard. Do you know why?

11

You think I'm going to have a fit.
No, I don't. But it could happen and
now that I know, it becomes awkward, legally.

I'm not going to have a fit. I never have them
when I feel good and the trapeze makes me
feel good, so I'm not going to have one
if I can use the trapeze.

She couldn't fault my logic.
Okay, she said as her hand
brushed her hair back off her face.
Don't upset yourself.

I'm not. It's everyone else
that's upsetting me.

Okay. I'm sorry. But let's see
if we can think this one through together.
I know that the trapeze means more to you
than anything else. That it means more to you
than perhaps to anyone else in this whole school.
I know you're good at it. And you're getting better.
But sometimes you're not very careful.
I've seen you in here by yourself without catchers.
That's dangerous for you.

How would you feel about using a safety belt?
I'd feel like a dog on a lead, I said.
She looked down and let out a hum of breath.
I looked down too.

Birds don't fly with leads, I said.
Safety belts are to learn with, not to live with . . .
just in case. I mean, Ms Quick, I'm safer on the
trapeze than crossing the road.
And I do that every day, often by myself.

She nodded. I'll talk to the Head and to Mrs Miller again.

I went home. Crossed the road. No cars ran me down.
No fits carried me away. I went home and sat
in the chair in front of the TV.
I couldn't get interested in dinner.
Mum tried to talk to me. But I wasn't worth talking to.
Anyway, she'd just agree with them.
I went to bed and finally cried.
Mum must have been standing at the door.
She came in a held me while I sobbed and sobbed.

They want to take it away from me, I wrenched out.
What do they want to take away?
The trapeze.
Why?
Mrs Miller saw me and she said I shouldn't be doing it
because of the fits. She told Ms Quick and said
it would be illegal for me to do it now that she,
Ms Quick, knows.
I said it wouldn't happen.
And I won't stop.

She said it would be illegal?
Mmm, she did.

Then Ms Quick said maybe I could
wear the safety belt all the time.
She almost brightened.
But, I said quickly, it wouldn't be the same.
I'd feel stupid. And everyone would wonder
why I suddenly started to use it.
Then they'd all make fun of me and tell one another
that it was because of the fits. Even though
I never have them at school. I don't want to be shackled.
I want to learn the trapeze like anyone else.
And Ms Quick says I'm good at it. Mum,
please don't tell them you think
the safety belt's a good idea.

xix
When the next class came round,
Gabriella had to wait for me.
I couldn't get my shoelaces tied up right.
What's with you?
Nothing.
Sure.

Ms Quick was at the other end talking
to a group of girls. The trapeze band
were already swinging around and laughing.
I stood in the door and watched. I could feel
prickles starting up in the corner of my eyes
and I turned my face into the fresh air.

She came over, took my shoulder
and guided me out the door.

Avis, I've worked something out.
You can do it, on one condition.
I listened as if my life depended on it. It did.
If I ever see you in here on your own,
without a catcher,
that's it.
She meant it.

I could hardly believe my luck.
They weren't going to ban me.
They weren't going to put me on a lead.
They were going to let me do it.
I nearly kissed her.

xx
I want to be a bird. And I will be.

THE LANGUAGE IN MY TONGUE

Enigma

Every day there are
Pills on the tongue
In the morning and at night.

Learning to cope,
Eventually it comes again—
Pillow wet, tongue bitten—

See the marks, the ridges—
Your teeth's tracks running
Evenly along one edge—

Pockets of blood. There's the
Interminable waiting; the
Living in the present,

Each day wondering, and you're
Pleased to have made it
So that tomorrow

You'll begin again. "Will it
Ever end?" you ask,
Pleading. Turning

Inward, you try to
Lead your mind another way,
Engaging in memories—

Prefabricated, imagined
Since only seen by others. For
You they are still too clear

Even though you were not
Present in a sense.
Inside, you know that

Living, simply living,
Establishing a routine,
Presents obstacle upon obstacle.

Safety is one thing,
Your independence another.
Equilibrium, plenty of sleep,

Patience, they all say—
Insensitive to your needs. Don't
Learn to drive, don't

Ever fly, or
Parachute, or scuba dive,
Since each could mean the end of

You. But what of life?
Epilepsy is not the end of it.
Pressures and stresses have an effect

Inevitably, then life goes on—
Living, loving like the rest,
Enjoying the world. You

Persist, sometimes you fail. You
Seem hardly affected by
Your fits. You wake

Each day to the
Possibility.
                              Once

I was there. You
Lunged towards the floor
Entered unconsciousness—

Pile of dancing muscles—
Slept until
Your eyes opened, blank

Empty. But you knew.
Perhaps it was my look.
It could have been the bruises

Left on your arms, your chin
Etched with a graze, a
Prickle of blood on your

Smooth tongue. "Sore,"
You said simply, stretching
Each limb as you

Perused the damage.
I felt powerless to help,
Longing to say something.

"Enigma" was the word that
Presented itself. A puzzle, but
Somehow the storms would pass.

Yawning, you came to again. Another
Electrical storm, another
Pulse of snapping synapses

Inching its way out slowly,
Leaving you thoroughly
Exhausted, leaving me

Perplexed at its
Suddenness and at
You.

Grand mal

I am an electrical impulse.
I dance.
I jump.
I leap across the abyss of the synapse.
I am an excessive and disorderly discharge.
I defy definition.
I recur from time to time.
I am random.
I am entirely cerebral.
I am at the threshold of a seizure.
Grand mal.
Idiopathic.
I give no warning.
I have no aura.
I leap from synapse to synapse.
I create disorder.
  She cries out.
I dance.
  She waves her arms about.
Everything is in a state of flux.
  She falls.
  Her pupils dilate.
  Her teeth bite into the tongue.
I am dancing.
  Her face is blue.
  Like the blue of cyanide.
I rampage.
I rage.
  Her muscles contract.
  She is seized.

She is prone.
She convulses.
Saliva dribbles from her mouth.
Saliva mixed with blood.
Her arms are bruised.
She is comatose.
She is unrousable.
She has lost consciousness.

The language of the serpent

There's a serpent in my head
growing wings.

How can I learn the grammar
of the serpent?

The pronouns, the particles, the
coiling syntax.

The language of the imaginary
reading

out from the centre
of the spiral—

The grammar of the
serpent language.

But the language of the serpent
is silent   still.

Transformation

She said to you:

I turned round to see what you
were staring at.
There was nothing.

That's when you fell.
When I wasn't watching.

When I turned back
your body was quivering,
shivering, shaking.

I don't know how long it lasted.
Two minutes or ten.

It felt like an hour.
I let you be. When you stopped
shaking, I held you.

It was a while before you woke.
Your eyes empty, not sparkling

as they usually do. They closed
again and inside some transformation
took place. When they opened again

they were alive. Then you slept,
breathing like a baby.

First breath

The first breath I took
was late.

I've been holding it ever since.

An amniotic sea pushing
me forwards.

But something was holding me back.

The doctor was late, so
I was too.

He breathed his lunch on me.

Words on mirrors

I write words on mirrors.
I begin with my blood.

My blood and words mix
creating a new syntax.

A syntax of relationships
between words and the self.

Something called reality.
Mine. Not theirs.

The reality of blood and words
that speak of other things.

There are eggs and words and worlds
and caves beneath the earth.

Susan Hawthorne

Miniature death

I dream of drowning
swimming upwards from the seabed
of unconsciousness.

My mouth opens
gasping for breath
like a fish near death.

I drown in my own held breath,
no water, no sea
just a miniature death.

In the bath

I confront my fear
               daily
sitting in twelve inches of water
                 in the bath

There are so many stories of fits in baths
that end with death
               by drowning

An eight year old child drowns
                 unsupervised for just a minute
An eighteen year old commits suicide
                 simply running the bath and waiting

I know it could happen
I've fallen often enough in the shower
only to wake to water-thinned
                 blood on my lips

I write this poem
               in my head
in twelve inches of water in the bath

24 hours

24 hours later I wake to the knowledge
        that slowly seeps through the
        labyrinthine passages
of another fit

24 hours only separates me from
        the knowledge of life and death

The bridge of my nose is bruised green
        my shoulder aches
        a finger in bone-bruised

The green monstera hanging over
        the bed where I lie
        quivers, its leaves shivering
in a vegetal seizure

Devils

Little devils with snarling carnivorous
mouths pursue me. Their teeth
sharp and furious, grip me
and I fall, damn it I fall . . .

Falling woman

I am the subject of my subject.
I fall.
I, the subject,
am subject to falling.

I fall in any old way.

I fall
sitting on a mattress
(the best way to fall)

I fall
sitting on a bicycle
sitting on a chair
sitting between people

I fall
standing in the shower
making a phone call

I fall
already lying down
sleeping in my bed

I fall in any old place

I fall
in bed with my lover
in the milk bar with unknown people
at home over breakfast
at work over my desk

I fall
in a meeting
in a hotel room
in a strange city

I am a woman who is
subject to falling.

Falling stars

I dissolve into a night
of falling stars.

Birds drop dead from
the sky.

I fall into night like the
dropping birds.

Wings lifted in a V as
they fall.

Winged arms stretched
to eternity.

Above, the stars
still fall.

No names

There are days when time falls away from me.
I cannot answer questions you put to me.
I have no words to answer with.

I see things.
I know there are names attached to the things.
I know I know them.
But the names are not there.

I have no name.
You have no name.
You are simply there.

Tongue without words

I have no words to answer with

words
     fall
         into the void
echoes
      empty
            of meaning
simple
      sounds
            stroking my waxy ears

I have no words to answer with

the tongue
        furled
           and hollow
the tongue
       grasping
           to feel meaning
the tongue
       flat
         out to speak

I have no words to answer with

the grey matter
         without
             static

no
  electrical charge
                 to spark meaning
no
  thing   to
               matter
no   thing   matters

nothing
     matters
I mutter
    something

something
      explodes
           in my brain

in my grey matter

something matters

my tongue
     stretches
         for the word
my tongue
     lifts
        presses against teeth
my tongue
     curls around a word

                        a hollow of meaning
a sound
        escapes
                the hollow curve of my mouth
a word
    I have a word
                    I have found the words
the words fall

            in a rush
                    spitting
                            frothing
words rush out
            filling the void

Black hole

> *for Sue*

Writing out of the black hole of a seizure.
I am another
      unfamiliar
even to myself.

My aching muscles
      arch.

My fingers clench a fist
      against some invisible
      other   self.

The muscles think first
      are in control
      long before I have
      returned to the grey cocoon.

The muscles are way ahead of the brain.

The muscles know how to drink coffee
      sipping mindlessly.
The cup is half empty
      and my brain has only just noticed.

Senseless

Unconscious and senseless,
threatening to swallow a
tongue full of words, all she could
do was gargle and gurgle with the
breath strangled in her throat.

Hyphen

I tense and the present dissolves.
Fuses short circuit in my brain.
Synapses cracked open are void.

There is blood on my lips.
Red lines on a page
depict my brain's circuit.

There's a hyphen between me
and the rest of the world,
breaking us apart.

My body is a country

My body is a country that I know.
Sometimes it dances under the moon.

I stretch my arms to reach for the
elusive thing I cannot see.

I kick up my feet, pillows of dust rise
and a branch caresses me as I pass.

My mouth opens and I call out to
the world around, weird sounds.

Red ants scuttle past my toes
as I dance.

Tongue

I am stiff.
My muscles ache
with inertia. My tongue

has blossomed in my mouth
            swelling.

There are holes
            ridges
            pockets of blood
            in my tongue.

My teeth puncture
the flesh of my tongue.
They bite into it.

The tongue bleeds.
The tongue
swells into bulkiness.

It swells and spreads
into all the cavities
of my mouth.

It does not feel like my tongue.

It is there
            hugely
            but it is as though it is not
                        a part of me.

Teeth

My tongue has been hacked at
with a blunt axe.

Teeth tear this succulent,
tender shaper of words.

The words fall off the tongue,
before speech can come.

The tongue swells with unspoken,
unshapeable words.

The words are swallowed
so that the tongue may remain

caught between teeth.

They thought you were dead

Someone said
They thought you were dead.

Later, she said
You fell like a rock
You didn't even bend your knees

Your colour was awful
You looked like you were dead
You didn't breathe for so long

Then, in a great rush
Air pulled itself into the vacuum of your lungs
Air filled the capillaries beneath the skin
Your face rushed red

You were so stiff
Muscles stretched and taut
As a bowstring
You were rigid

Later, she said
You lay so still
So quiet
I thought maybe you were dead after all.

Dying stars

I don't remember what went before.
There was a river rising, a lake
that spread itself across the paddock
before the sun rose.

There was waking to the thunderous sound
of a river breaking banks and
watching the sun rise over still
water that lay all around.

There was a magazine, an article
about the death of stars, of the
gravitational pull of inhuman
forces, annihilation.

There was the gravitational pull of
earthly forces, pulling me towards
a human death, annihilating
my will to rise.

There was simple blackness, void.

Underworld

The gods have me again—
they lift me high and
hurl me into the chasm

I lie there struggling to
breathe, but they have no
mercy, they trample me

beneath hob-nailed boots,
the underworld beckons,
their little hands seizing

me, dragging me down to
earth's maw.
          Someone

takes pity, levers me upwards
towards the light. Do not look
back, she says. Do not ask

what happened, just step
forward
        into the light

Eurydice

Orpheus sings as he returns
from the dead.

Eurydice cries out, Don't
leave me here like this.

Eurydice's eyes are dry
with fear and anger

As darkness closes in on her
once again.

Dream moon

for Renate

In a dream
      in some kind of fit or seizure
      that lasted three days
      your memory vanished.

Dream memory.
Dream moon.

      A day the parakeet, red with sailing suns
      stretched her wings across the orb
      of that blinding light.

Dream moon.
Dream memory.

      A time when black cockatoos screeched and
      the moon rose yellow and red against black
      like tail feathers.

In a dream
      there was only you, and her
      screeching like cockies on a bare tree.

In some kind of fit or seizure
      there was blackness, a void.

And only later
      there was the sun shining into your
      upturned eyes, still closed.

Red.
And yellow.
And black.

In a dream
      in some kind of fit or seizure
      these things happened.

New tongue

You say that later
they said that when your memory failed
you recognised only your sister
your companion.

You say some thought you were dead.

But when, after three days you woke.
Your ears heard the world as if for the first time.
Your eyes saw the white cockatoo long before she flew over
dropping feathers on your head.

You sang in a new tongue
or so others said.
You picked up a large stick brandishing it at all
except your sister your companion.

You say that in your dream
            in some kind of fit or seizure
            you were entrusted with language.

Susan Hawthorne

The well

Women meet at the well head—
They are perched high above me
their faces black against
the bright blue of the sky

I rest deep in the well
as they toss orphan words
into the depths, waiting
for the plink, calculating the depth.

Oracle

The words escape me,
I grasp at them, wordlessly,
lava flows in rivers
through me, turning
my life to ash
burning every bridge
I cross, I turn
and watch them collapse.

Out of ashes two figures
rise, silhouetted against
the flaming sky—
phoenix-like they rise,
slowly, rise and rise again,
rising in great arched waves,
until the tsunami crashes
on to the shore.

There she stands,
her mouth opening
words frothing, words
rushing out in riddles
that only sphinxes and
oracles understand . . .

Words caught on the
tongue's breath,
words slipping silently

from mouths like
spittled fingers,
words carrying me
away, wingéd words . . .

The language in my tongue

My tongue has blossomed in my mouth
It is filled with language
It spreads like a big red balloon
With language caught inside

A language that can't distinguish one thing from another
A language that does not care for past or future
A language tense with the present

The language in my tongue dissolves all history
It dissolves all expectation of the future
The language in my tongue is a big red balloon

There's a language in my body too
A language in the arch of my back
A language in the froth from my mouth
A language in my clenched fist
A language in the cry from my lungs
There's a language in my bleeding tongue

The language in my body and in my tongue
is the language they spoke in Delphi.
The language of the seizure that dispels time,
that defies death, that returns the orator
to the world of light, that single point that
draws me back from the inertia, the gravity
field of a hole so black, nothing exists
and nothing matters.

Susan Hawthorne

Eyes

Nothing matters
except the eyes you wake to

brown eyes
blue eyes
adult eyes
child eyes

eyes that ask questions
for which you have no answers.

Eyes matter.

The skin on my tongue

We make love in the afternoon.
It is hot and it is with
tears and grief for our unmourned
losses that we come together.

The heat settles on us as we sleep.
You so deeply that you do not feel
the bed shake. I wake, my fingers
clenched, my muscles aching.

It is hours before I realise. Cleaning
my teeth that night, the toothpaste stings
the broken skin on my tongue. I say,
I must have had another fit.

Traces

Traces of footprints in earth.
Traces in time.
Traces meeting and parting.
A network of lines.

They resemble the tracks
        left by sheep
        or electrons
        or red ink on a page.

EEG

I try to listen to my body.
Like a seismograph, I attend to
the quakes and eruptions.

In the hospital with its electro-
encephalograph, I watch the recording
of my brain's electrical storms.

The nurse begins with the conductive
jelly, rubbed cold into my scalp,
electrodes and a rubber cap.

I'm all wired up and connected
to the machine. The switch is flicked to on
and the machine is off and running

red tracks across pages, making
mountain peaks of alpha waves, beta
waves and others I cannot name.

I open and close my eyes on command.
The machine hums on. Sometimes
a strobe is placed, like a giant sun,

in front of my face. Mandalas flash.
Hallucinations retreat in circles.
Kaleidoscopes spin and I smile.

Strobe

There is a big flashing sun
       orange and blue
       red and green
       purple and yellow

flashing as though the world
       were ready to end

close your eyes
           open your eyes
                     green
             flashes
         red

open your eyes
           close your eyes
                   purple
             flashes
        yellow

close your eyes
           open your eyes
                  orange
             flashes
       blue

There are a thousand suns
       all falling one upon the other

A thousand suns my eyes are trying
      to avoid

But a thousand suns up against your nose
      is there even if you

close your eyes
              open your eyes
                  to see it

Concrete words

There are words
        as heavy as concrete
        falling.

There are words
        bright and gleaming and sharp
        as steel.

A word pierces my skull
        like a nail shattering
        bone.

Insects compose songs
        hanging from leaves in the
        summer night air.

Flowers paint the trees
        in mauve and yellow and
        splashes of red.

Red and green paint
        spatter the concrete
        words.

Sixteen years

Sixteen years
    from one fit to the next

I thought
    maybe

It wouldn't happen again

But it did.

The flood

for Primrose

When the flood came and I was twenty
it began again.

My father strapped himself to the tree and slept above
the swirling water.

He came home in a boat with men in yellow raincoats
carrying sandwiches.

The next day I fell from my chair
at breakfast.

My mother, believing ancient advice, pressed her finger
into my mouth.

In unconsciousness I bit, into bone
which cracked.

Now, when her finger hurts, she knows
a cold change is coming.

When I woke, I slept again. I felt
battered, beaten.

For three days I slept and woke, woke
and slept again.

Afterwards, we drove the tractor along the
cracked bitumen road.

Slabs of road angled where the earth had
expanded into clay.

My mother and I walked along the river as it fell back
into its banks.

She said, That day, I thought you had died.
Better my finger.

Sometimes I think I did, a part of me died in
those three days:

I lost my belief in immortality.

Susan Hawthorne

Ransom

for Dale

i
I am held in ransom for life—
and terror covers my head
like a balaclava—
only the eyes stare out.

Death shoves me from behind,
I turn but cannot see death's
face in this dark corner.

It hauls me across the room,
head banging against the tiled
floor, there is a dull thud
of a body falling.

Legs kick against kitchen
cupboards. Like a fish out
of water, the mouth gasps
in an agony of helplessness.

ii
Life sidles up to me,
I sit up, stare   disoriented.
You cajole me into sense.

Restless as a rabbit, I scurry
about the room until men
in blue uniforms arrive with
an ambulance to take me away—

No, I say, and No again
standing my ground against
medical reason.

Life and death push me around.

Relearning the language caught inside my tongue

Mother, help me!
Help me return from my death.
Draw the blood back to my face.
Push air into my lungs.
Mother, help me!

Mother, help me!
Fold my legs across your arms.
Still the quaking muscles.
Silence the terror in my eyes.
Mother, help me!

Mother, help me!
Return to me the words they've taken.
Colour my memory with images.
Invent a history for me.
Mother, help me!

Mother, help me!
The trees are pulling my body apart.
The fabric of my mind is crushed.
The sun is cutting out my eyes.
Mother, help me!

Help me relearn the language
caught inside my tongue.

Belly language

My language is the language of the woman
who has fallen, comatose, a slight

entity, thin as twigs on a tree, her skin
wrinkling like the bark in the bend

of a eucalypt. My language is the language
of the hot stone, still

and too hot to touch, smoothed round
by time. My language is the language

of the hills folding, the kaltu-kaltu
bending in the wind across the desert.

My language is the language of the caves
that collapse into the earth,

the limestone drip that builds fantastic cities
underground, some hanging and never

breaking. My language is the language
of the river that meanders, cutting

its soft body into hard rock. My language
is the language of the belly.

Susan Hawthorne

ECT

How would you feel if your body
gave you a spontaneous ECT?

Thesaurus

Epilepsy
>   see *spasm*
>   *frenzy*
>   *nervous disorders*

Embedded near spasm are: convulsion and orgasm
                                  fit and seizure
under the general heading of **Agitation**

I find frenzy under the general heading of **Insanity**
>   only a semi-colon or two separates me from
>   *alcoholism*
>   *unintelligibility*
>   *hysteria*
and a variety of manias

I wonder why it wasn't placed instead under
>   **Oblivion**, blankness

I search for nervous disorders
>   *psychopathy*
>   *insensibility*
>   *spasm*
Here at last: petit mal, grand mal, epilepsy, falling sickness

And this is the New Edition!

Suggestions for a new thesaurus:
Epilepsy

see	**Religion**	sacred disease, falling sickness, epilepsy, ecstasy
	Unconsciousness	blankness, forgetfulness, Lethe, oblivion, confusion, black hole
	Spasm	seizure, convulsion, muscular agitation, grand mal, petit mal, fit
	Illness	status epilepticus, accidental injury, breathlessness, ECT

SEIZED

Variations on Sappho's Fragment 31

i

To me you are divine
as you play your role—
speaking, listening,
laughing that laugh

running through me
like an electric current.
The shock, the jolt as I
watch. My voice

dries up; it is hot like sand
in a desert creekbed
and it slides slowly away
from me. My eyes die,

I hear nothing as
lava flows under
my skin. Seized,
my mind flees—

down, down into the
underworld, into a
kind of death.

ii
Fortune has deserted me today
as I watch the one sitting
face to face with you

Across the room I listen as
words and laughter fall
from your lips

My heart becomes a
jolting carriage and my
tongue is electrified by

fear. Fire runs through
my veins and I can no longer
hear your words, your laughter,

for the humming in my ears.
I convulse, and sweat
runs cool down my face,

pale as summer-dried grass—
death would be better
than this jealousy.

iii
I watch her, your public face;
I hear her speak the expected words
of coupling love.

Her smile eats at me like acid;
my ribs are scorched and the
heart jolts inside its cage.

When I look at you, heart
emptied, voice hollowed,
now meaningless

I speak empty breath.
My tongue fallow, no
harvest of words

only froth, a dead-eyed
gaze and muscles that
cringe convulsively.

My mind quivers, retreats
toward death, and I know
that only death is an end.

i

Endnote

Sappho. Fragment 31.

There has been centuries of discussion about Fragment 31, and re-reading it one night it hit me that the poem could be about the experience of an epileptic seizure. The descriptions of bodily sensations are not too dissimilar, and so I decided to write a poem with that in mind. I finished up with three variations. For those unfamiliar with this poem of Sappho, I am reproducing a translation by Gillian Spraggs.

This version translated by Gillian Spraggs in "Divine Visitations: Sappho's Poetry of Love". Elaine Hobby and Chris White. (Eds.) 1991. *What Lesbians Do in Books*. London: The Women's Press, p. 55. Of all the translations I have read of this poem, Gillian Spraggs' translation seems to pick up the subtleties best. Here is her version.

He seems to me the peer of gods, that man
who sits and faces you,
close by you hearing
your sweet voice speaking,

and your sexy laugh, which just this moment makes
the heart quake in my breast: for every time
I briefly glance towards you, then I lose
all power of further speech.

My tongue is smashed; at once a film of fire
runs underneath my skin; no image shapes
before my eyes;
my ears are whining like a whirling top;

cold sweat pours down me, and in every part
shuddering grips me;
I am paler than summer grass,
and seem to myself to be at the point of death.

TONGUE TIED

Hilda's journey

Hilda plays roulette with her life.
She has explored the
Amazon basin and Egypt's crypts.
Alone she crept
through darkened labyrinths. Her
journey is almost over.

Tomorrow she will leave with the
rising sun and pass
beyond the horizon. In preparation
she grits her teeth
and holds death's violets therein.

The improbable city

I dreamt of a city built on water,
where walls reached for the sky,
and a boat with one oar sailed silently.

I dreamt of a city where people wore
masks for one day a year. A day when
no one knew who stood next to them.

I dreamt of an artist who painted
clocks like water, where one-oared
boats carrying masked people drifted.

I dreamt of a woman who fell face
forward on the ground, frothing
blood and speaking incantations.

I dreamt of a place where hot sand was
blown into the shape of a galloping
horse, coloured and translucent.

I dreamt of a place where the
improbable happened daily and
the people sat and drank and watched.

Year's end

Mountains curved white, rising
perpendicular rock above the water,
flat blue.

The path winds its way around
the lapping edge, sometimes passing
through solid rock.

No one wants to know you on the
last day of the year, when the snow
lies thick.

Only old friends are welcome to eat
by the fire. So you travel to the end
of the lake.

Yesterday you brushed past death,
galloping faster this time, although your head
lay in the snow.

Birds are few. Black against the white.
They sit in leafless trees or follow sheep
as they graze.

Returning, the full moon dogs our
path, fingering shadowed rock, creating
pools of light.

Unripe

Unripe virgin oil,
mastigia and pith of the lotus
boiled with marjoram—

So said the ancients—
a cure for possession
by vile daemons.

And words chanted
in the ears of the
frothing-mouthed one:

"Lift this one, our sister,
out of darkness,
come, lift her head—

Bind the thoughts
separated like beads
on a string—

Return from death,
oh great listless one—
arise, arise!"

Gone

She has gone,
her death as fast as her life

Gone in an explosion
of electrical current, burning bright

as she descends
into the underworld behind consciousness

She has gone
silent in her wide bed, her tongue

hacked by teeth,
the body injuring itself in its last

attempt to seize life,
seized death by mistake

She is gone
and no amount of electricity,

run through brain
and heart, will bring her back.

Susan Hawthorne

Hell and back

If the cells in the body
remember every act
every fall into the void

then I've been to hell
and back a dozen times.

Tongue tied

The tongue is pushed back
into a curl, the flesh

slit from beneath and,
as the knot of tongue

curls back further into
speech, she cries out:

"Tell me what you know,
tell me again, over and over,

so that I will know it
in my bones and in my belly,

in my ears and in my mouths,
so that I may speak it with

my unknotted tongue,
and it will come out of me

like blood, like spittle,
like trembling tears."

The pot

words a fracture a crack in a pot
                                a pot with
words inscribed on its surface
                        a vision of a novel written
            on the surface of
                a pot
                a three dimensional novel
                how else to write a novel
        in these post-modernist days? the novel
has a unique structure
        the structure of the pot
        the structure of the fracture
                    the fracture occurs in
            the side of the pot it shivers its way from
        the rim to
                    the base
                        it is not deep enough to crack
                        it
                    the fracture makes the pot fragile
        the scribe must work with utmost care
like the artist who carves designs on the eggs of emus
    the scribe,
also the writer, is a woman, she
                    is inventing a new world by writing
                        on the fractured egg-pot
                            the egg breaks and out of
        it is formed the world
                    the world   egg
                    the woman fashions a pot from
    clay

the clay formed
        by the world   egg
           she leaves the pot and in
        time a fracture appears
          the fracture gives rise to symbols
characters
    hieroglyphs
        ideographs
words   she inscribes
words on to the pot
       she writes a novel on the surface
  of the pot
      the pot is
cracked
            a fracture
words

No witness

To be no witness
to an event
experienced in the
body, absent from
the mind.

The tongue is the
only witness
I have to nocturnal
fits, slept through—
not woken from.

The broken tongue
speaks silent words
in the shreds of
skin that sting
and ache.

As the day proceeds
I begin to wonder,
puzzled I run my
finger along the
ridged edge.

Still not believing
I stand in front
of the mirror
stretching to see
the teeths' marks.

Unconvinced, I
want a witness,
though the body
shows its experience
I am no witness to it.

Microlandscapes

There are landscapes in the brain, nerve and muscle
forming rivers. A delta of canals and cytoplasmic fields
bordered by bushland. Billabongs and salt pans dot
the landscape—a microlandscape we carry within us.
Inner landscapes imitating the world outside.

Synapse

The synapse is caught in the nannomoment of firing
little lights, dancing along the edge of the myelin sheath
dancing as if someone's life depended on the dance.

The synapse is firing and something is wrong
impulses shoot randomly, scattering through the body,
not travelling the arterial route to headquarters.

The synapse is firing and I am falling, like a star
hurtling through space, I am falling into an infinite
void of millions of nannomoments.

The synapse is firing, firing, firing
the impulses glowing, phosphorescent, incandescent,
firing, firing, firing.

The synapse is firing and I have fallen, body shaking
with synaptic quivers, the mouth is gargling mangled sounds,
the legs kicking, arms thrashing—and the synapse is firing.

Starfish

Like a starfish, floating
I free fall
into the vortex.

Little lights glimmer,
phosphorescent
across the waves.

Diamond crystals in a cave
winking in the flash
of my camera.

A body stilled by capturing
light through the lens
of a black box.

Stilled in movement—
light flashes out across
aeons of void.

Fear creases through eyes
as awareness returns
to this face.

Like a starfish, light
crystallises in eyes
which gaze into the lens.

I saw eternity

i
I saw eternity
and it was coloured bright
acid etched into the walls

iridescent phantoms
caressing with seductive
breath, speaking

with my mouth—
"I can die," I said,
and promptly went on living.

ii
I saw eternity
and it was of no colour at all,
darkness throttled me,

etched in electrical pulses,
an invisible wall—
the void called me,

scrambled words as it passed by,
its warm breath
removing all the words

from my mouth—
I fell into gibberish
and the littleness of a miniature death.

MEDITATION ON FALLING

What is the velocity of a falling body?   a body moving through space, sensing neither the relative time, nor the relative motion of its fall.

How long does a body   falling into a seizure   take to fall?

Which is the time?
Which is the space?

If a body is senseless to the motion the time the space the pull of gravity as she falls   can she be a sentient body?

If a body only notices that she has fallen (now face down on the ground)   that it happened some time before this moment   (her eyes open to her position but not to any memory)   that gravity has pulled her down   how can she know she has fallen?   that time itself has been seized?   that memory has not encoded the moment or the actualisation of the fall?   What then?

If memory has for a moment   (or for several unquantifiable moments)   been erased scrubbed clean by the fall through time through space   what proof has she that she exists?

Only later, when she says   What happened?   (assuming something did)   can she call on her existence. But when she fell sensing none of the things essential to conscious existence   did she exist as anything more than an object falling?

She can know only that she has fallen through space into another time   but only as an object.   At the moment of non-existence she cannot be a subject (except that she is subject to the laws of gravity and the continuous flow of space/time).

At the moment of non-existence during the fall   she   (like any particle)   could move along one of two paths   a tendency towards non-existence   (death)   in which case the subjectless state would have persisted   or she could resonate towards a tendency to exist   (which she did)   and move back towards the possibility of subjectivity.

She leaves a frail trail of light   burning brighter   as consciousness returns to her eyes.

She lives!

Susan Hawthorne

THE ADVENTURES OF AN EPILEPTIC

*You never know what strange adventures are going to befall you
when you have epilepsy. You meet people in the strangest places
and the strangest ways.*

i

Eyes. Brown. Blue. Brown again.
Shoulders. Some stooping. Some straight.
The eyes staring. Staring through you.

No one you recognise. Standing over you.
A woman. An old woman. An old woman in black.
Close. Very close to you. Brown eyes.

She strokes you with her hand. Speaking in riddles.
You hear the birds singing in Greek. Ela. Ela.

A room. Strange. Full of boxes. Coloured boxes.
You search. Your eyes roaming. But what are you searching for?
Grappling with nothingness.

Wet. Where is the wetness from? Lying in water. Why?
The old woman in black. Her eyes and children's x-ray eyes.
Lying in a pool of water. The eyes talk. The old woman strokes.

Who are they? Who is she? Who are you?

You turn your head into cold water.
Spaghetti. Toilet rolls. Cat food.
Your head flat against the concrete floor.

The eyes mill above you. The fog is in your mind.
The old woman again. She pulls at you. Pulls you to sitting.
A door opens to the street. Coloured plastic strips in the wind.

Children tangled in green, orange, yellow, blue, red strips.
Beyond the door. Dark. At the other end a counter.
Ice-cream cones. An unused milkshake maker.

The old woman smiles. Her face as crinkled as the paper bags.
A milk bar. The old woman points to the door. Eyes follow her
hand. A familiar face. But nameless. Bustles through the door.

You are lifted. Arms around shoulders.
You turn toward the old woman in black. Want to say thank you.
For caring. For holding your hand. No words. Only eyes.

You sleep heavily. No dreams. Like the sleep of the dead.

The milk bar looms large when you wake. Must say something.
The old woman in black stands behind the counter.
Despina. Despina. Ela, she calls.

Hello. How are you today? Better? Yes, I'm okay now, thanks.
Has it happened before? Yes. Yes, it has.
But not in a milk bar, you think.

Anna is not unusual. She's a student. An activist. She attends
meetings, goes to dances. Has a good time.

ii
At the Rape Crisis Centre meeting you discuss strategies
Six women deciding who should go to the court committal.
Text book case. A lane off Bourke Street. He's on bail.

When's it on?" asks Jane. Your arms are raised and you gaze
blank-eyed. Jane tosses a box of matches. Hey, dreamy,
when's it on? You fall, knocking knuckles against the brick wall.

Jane leaps to your side. Oh, god, what've I done?
Looks to me like she having a fit, says Sarah calmly.
I knew a girl at school who had them.

What do we do? I don't know.
Why don't we call Lisa? offers Wendy, she'll know what to do.
Jane cradles your head in her lap.

I thought I'd knocked her out, Jane says to no one in particular.
It missed her, says Julie. I thought what a good shot.
But she was already out by then.

*Some people just don't get it. Some people think you've knocked
your head and fallen unconscious. Well, I don't suppose you can
blame them—it's not always the first explanation that comes to
mind.*

iii

The bicycle lies in the centre of the road, quivering.
By the time neighbours reach you, you are still.
The bicycle too—except for the mad spinning of its back wheel.

I hope she hasn't got concussion, says Mr Bernardino.
I don't fancy spending the day at Out Patients.
Mrs Bernadino makes coffee. Her eyes are glassy, she says.

Now dear, drink this, the coffee should make you feel better.
That was a nasty fall you took. You nod.
Where'd this coffee come from? How'd I get here? What fall?

What fall? you ask. You fell off your bike. Don't you remember?
No. I don't know these people. I wonder where I am?
They think I know them. But I don't. You look at the coffee.

The coffee's half gone. What happened?
I don't remember getting on my bike, let alone falling off it. Shit.
I suppose they saw me fall and assumed I'd knocked myself out.

Did your foot miss the pedal? asks Mrs Bernardino. Maybe.
Probably too many late nights—you shouldn't study so late.
Well, I'd better go, I'm already late. Late for what, you wonder.

You're surprised to see your house is next door.
I just have to get a few things. You rummage through your bag
to find out where you're going.

Sometimes you find yourself in places you wouldn't have predicted. You can finish up being with other strange women.

iv
You wake to a strange bed. Your mind blank. Empty.
A woman bends over you, half naked.
Do you remember anything of last night?

No. That's a pity, it was such a good night.
I know you, but I can't remember your name. Rosemary.
Rosemary. And me? You're Anna.

Emptiness presses you back against the sheet.
Silence. You try to find an order to the chaos in your mind.
Try to fill the blank spaces with something substantial.

You came to dinner. Did I drink too much?
Yes. Does that make a difference? It seems to.
Something stirs in the empty blackness inside your head.

An image here and there that you can barely grasp.
Rosemary takes you through the sequence. A jigsaw.
Scattered pieces of unrelated patterns gradually join up.

It is slow. Painstaking. And some confusion persists.
You have no memory of waking. But you have a yesterday.
Yellow sunlight envelops Rosemary. Like a Russian icon.

I was too slow to put something in your mouth, she says.
Not a good idea. Better just to hold the person.
I always bite my tongue anyway. See.

It's not just strange houses you find yourself in. It's strange predicaments.

v

You wake, wallowing in the sun. You open your eyes.
Another unfamiliar room. It must have happened again.
You sit up in bed and look out over the harbour. Sydney?

You try to think. How did you get there?
You flop back on the pillows.
I'll ring home. No. Can't do that.

Can't remember the phone number.
There must be a telephone book here.
Hello. Melbourne. Poloni. Fitzroy. Thank you.

Hello. I think I've had a fit. I'm in Sydney, but I can't remember
why or how long I've been here, or where I am in Sydney.
I think I'm in a hotel . . . All right. You'll ring me back?

You doze. Waiting. But no call comes.
You get out of bed. No bag. Nothing in the cupboard.
Nothing in the drawers. No books beside the bed.

You go back to bed. Pulling the cover up.
A dawning suspicion creeps through your brain.
They have to find me. Can't go out naked.

Time dawdles by. A knock. Come in, you say.
The sheets to your chin. I seem to be in the wrong room.
Are you all right? asks the housekeeper.

This is room 805. You're booked into 807.
Back in 807, the phone rings.
I must have walked along the corridor naked.

*You get used to the unfamiliar places and after a while you learn
to devise ways of working out where you are. It takes a lot of
stamina not to panic.*

vi
The silence gets to you. Mad epileptics. Spectacular fits.
The brother, the friend the daughter, the lover who died
in bed, in the bath, in a motorcycle accident.

Do we all die like that? No warning?
Just an end? A never returning to consciousness?
You'd rather die conscious.

You have a sense of having returned from death.
Emerging from the void. It's not like sleep, there are no dreams
to people the silence with. It is an unscaleable inertia.

Acknowledgements

The translation from Greek of Sappho's Fragment 31 is by Gillian Spraggs in "Divine Visitations: Sappho's Poetry of Love" in Elaine Hobby and Chris White. (Eds.) 1991. *What Lesbians Do in Books*. London: The Women's Press, p. 55. Reprinted with kind permission from the translator.

The sequence, "The Language in My Tongue" was previously published in the collection, *Four New Poets* (Penguin Books, 1993). Poems from that sequence have been published in the *Age*, *Fine Line*, *Meanjin*, *Time Magazine* (Australia), *Slow Dancer* (UK), *Tessera* (Canada), *Sinister Wisdom* (USA), and in the following books: Jillian Bartlett and Cathi Joseph. (Eds.) 1991. *Body Lines*. Sydney: Women's Redress Press; Paul Kavanagh. (Ed.) 1991. *The Sea's White Edge*. Springwood, NSW: Butterfly Books; Susan Hawthorne. 1992. *The Falling Woman*. Spinifex Press. Nine poems also appear in Neil Buchanan. 1994. *Understanding Epilepsy*. Sydney: Simon and Schuster.

"The pot" was first published in Irene Coates, Nancy J. Corbett and Barbara Petrie. (Eds.) 1987. *Up From Below*. Sydney: Women's Redress Press.

"The adventures of an epileptic" was first published in a different form in *Sinister Wisdom 39: On Disability*. Winter 1989–90.

"Meditation on falling" was first published in Roberta Snow and Jill Taylor. (Eds.) 1993. *Falling for Grace*. Sydney: Blackwattle Press.

"I saw eternity" was first published in Sue Goss. (Ed.) 1995. *Epilepsy: I Can Live With That*. Melbourne: Epilepsy Foundation of Victoria.

"Seized" was first published in Diane Bell and Renate Klein. (Eds.) 1996. *Radically Speaking: Feminism Reclaimed*. Melbourne: Spinifex Press.

"Bird" (in a slightly different form) was Highly Commended in the National FAW Lyn Simmonds Award, 1996.
"The Flood" was shortlisted in the Mattara Poetry Awards, 1991.